HEART DISEASE DIET COOKBOOK FOR SENIORS

20 Flavorful Recipes With Low-Salt And Low-Fat For a Healthier Lifestyle

Rebecca Dorron

Table Of Contents

Introduction

Meet Jane, a lively senior who found herself at a crossroads when confronted with heart health problems. Determined to take responsibility, she found the "Heart Disease Diet Cookbook for Seniors." What began as a simple improvement to her kitchen rapidly became a guidebook to restoring her energy.

Jane enjoyed the cookbook's numerous recipes, from tasty fish meals to comforting vegetable stews. Each meal became a celebration of food, a symphony of colors and sensations that connected with her taste senses and her emotions. The cookbook's focus on nutritious grains, lean meats, and antioxidant-rich fruits and vegetables became the cornerstone of her daily decisions.

As the weeks progressed, Jane sensed a difference. Her energy levels increased, and the scale started to show a fresh equilibrium. Regular check-ups indicated good decreases in her lipid levels and blood pressure. The cookbook wasn't simply a compilation of recipes; it became a companion in her quest to manage and even reverse her heart health difficulties.

Today, Jane is not only eating excellent meals; she's appreciating life. The "Heart Disease Diet Cookbook for Seniors" became her ally, turning the page into a healthy, heart-happy chapter in her senior years. After all, age is only a number, and Jane is living evidence that a well-curated cookbook may be the formula for a heart-healthy and enjoyable existence. Cheers to excellent meals and a healthier heart!

Managing heart disease is an important journey, and a heart-focused diet may be a great ally. A specialized "Heart Disease Diet Cookbook" provides more than recipes; it's a guide to wellbeing. Packed with heart-smart options – from omega-3 rich fish to antioxidant-loaded fruits – it converts meals into a defense against cardiovascular difficulties. With each mouthful, the cookbook inspires consumers to take charge of their health. It's not just about tastes; it's a strategic approach to supporting the heart, converting dietary choices into a proactive stand against heart disease. A recipe becomes a daily medicine for a heart-healthy existence.

THIS PAGE WAS INTENTIONALLY LEFT BLANK

Mouthwatering And Delicious Recipes

1. Salmon with Lemon-Dill Sauce

INTRODUCTION:
A heart-healthy meal rich in omega-3 fatty acids. Salmon supports cardiovascular well-being, and the tangy lemon-dill sauce offers a rush of taste.

INGREDIENTS:
- Salmon fillets
- Fresh lemon juice
- Fresh dill, chopped
- Olive oil
- Garlic, minced
- Salt and pepper

PREPARATION METHOD:
1. Preheat oven to 375°F (190°C).

2. Place fish on a baking sheet.

3. Mix lemon juice, chopped dill, olive oil, minced garlic, salt, and pepper in a bowl.

4. Brush the mixture over fish.

5. Bake for 15-20 minutes or until fish is flaky.

2. Quinoa and Vegetable Stir-Fry

INTRODUCTION:

Loaded with fiber and antioxidants, this quinoa stir-fry is a tasty and heart-friendly alternative for seniors. Packed with colorful vegetables for extra nutrition.

INGREDIENTS:

- Quinoa, cooked
- Broccoli florets
- Carrots, julienned
- Bell peppers, sliced
- Low-sodium soy sauce

- Sesame oil
- Ginger, grated
- Garlic, minced

PREPARATION METHOD:

1. In a wok, stir-fry broccoli, carrots, and bell peppers.
2. Add cooked quinoa to the veggies.
3. Mix low-sodium soy sauce, sesame oil, grated ginger, and chopped garlic in a bowl.
4. Pour the sauce over the quinoa and veggies.
5. Stir until completely blended.

3. Oven-Baked Chicken Breast with Herbs

INTRODUCTION:

A lean protein choice to assist heart health. Oven-baked chicken breasts seasoned with heart-protective herbs make for a quick and healthy supper.

INGREDIENTS:
- Chicken breasts
- Fresh rosemary and thyme, chopped
- Olive oil
- Garlic powder
- Lemon zest
- Salt and pepper

PREPARATION METHOD:
1. Preheat oven to 400°F (200°C).
2. Rub chicken breasts with chopped rosemary, thyme, olive oil, garlic powder, lemon zest, salt, and pepper.
3. Bake for 25-30 minutes or until chicken is cooked through.

4. Mediterranean Chickpea Salad

INTRODUCTION:
A refreshing and fiber-rich salad incorporating chickpeas, recognized for their heart-boosting effects. This

Mediterranean-inspired recipe is loaded with nutrition.

INGREDIENTS:
- Canned chickpeas, rinsed
- Cherry tomatoes, halved
- Cucumber, diced
- Red onion, coarsely chopped
- Feta cheese, crumbled
- Kalamata olives, sliced
- Olive oil
- Red wine vinegar
- Oregano, dried
- Salt and pepper

PREPARATION METHOD:
1. In a bowl, mix chickpeas, cherry tomatoes, cucumber, red onion, feta cheese, and Kalamata olives.
2. In a separate dish, mix together olive oil, red wine vinegar, dried oregano, salt, and pepper.
3. Pour the dressing over the chickpea mixture.

4. Toss until nicely coated.

5. Spinach and Berry Salad with Walnut Vinaigrette

INTRODUCTION:
Packed with antioxidants, this salad combines the heart-healthy benefits of spinach, berries, and walnuts. The walnut vinaigrette provides a delicious nutty taste.

INGREDIENTS:
- Fresh spinach leaves
- Mixed berries (strawberries, blueberries, raspberries)
- Walnuts, chopped
- Olive oil
- Balsamic vinegar
- Dijon mustard
- Honey
- Salt & pepper

PREPARATION METHOD:

1. In a large bowl, combine fresh spinach, mixed berries, and chopped walnuts.
2. In a small bowl, mix together olive oil, balsamic vinegar, Dijon mustard, honey, salt, and pepper.
3. Drizzle the vinaigrette over the salad.
4. Toss lightly to coat.

6. Baked Sweet Potatoes with Cinnamon

INTRODUCTION:

Sweet potatoes, rich in fiber and beta-carotene, form a heart-healthy side dish. Baked to perfection with a sprinkling of cinnamon for a hint of sweetness.

INGREDIENTS:

- Sweet potatoes, peeled and cubed
- Olive oil

- Cinnamon
- Salt

PREPARATION METHOD:
1. Preheat oven to 400°F (200°C).
2. Toss diced sweet potatoes with olive oil, cinnamon, and salt.
3. Spread them on a baking sheet in a single layer.
4. Bake for 25-30 minutes or until sweet potatoes are cooked.

7. Mushroom and Spinach Stuffed Chicken Breast

INTRODUCTION:
Lean chicken breast meets the richness of mushrooms and the healthiness of spinach in this wonderful recipe. High in protein and low in fat, it's a heart-healthy and tasty option.

INGREDIENTS:

- Chicken breasts
- Mushrooms, chopped
- Fresh spinach leaves
- Garlic, minced
- Low-sodium chicken broth
- Olive oil
- Thyme, dried
- Salt and pepper

PREPARATION METHOD:

1. Preheat oven to 375°F (190°C).

2. Sauté chopped mushrooms and minced garlic in olive oil until soft.

3. Add fresh spinach and simmer until wilted.

4. Butterfly chicken breasts and fill with the mushroom and spinach mixture.

5. Place packed chicken breasts in a baking tray.

6. Pour low-sodium chicken stock over the chicken.

7. Sprinkle with dried thyme, salt, and pepper.

8. Bake for 25-30 minutes or until chicken is cooked through.

8. Lentil and Vegetable Soup

INTRODUCTION:
A hearty and heart-protective soup including lentils and an assortment of veggies. Packed with fiber and minerals, it's a soothing and healthful alternative.

INGREDIENTS:
- Brown lentils, washed
- Carrots, diced
- Celery, chopped
- Onion, finely chopped
- Garlic, minced
- Low-sodium vegetable broth
- Tomatoes, diced
- Bay leaves
- Cumin, ground

- Coriander, ground
- Salt and pepper

PREPARATION METHOD:

1. In a large saucepan, sauté onion, garlic, carrots, and celery until softened.

2. Add brown lentils, diced tomatoes, vegetable broth, bay leaves, ground cumin, ground coriander, salt, and pepper.

3. Bring to a boil, then decrease heat and simmer until lentils are cooked.

4. Remove bay leaves before serving.

9. Garlic and Herb Roasted Vegetables

INTRODUCTION:

Colorful and nutrient-packed, these roasted veggies are seasoned with heart-healthy garlic and herbs. A delightful side dish that compliments any heart-conscious dinner.

INGREDIENTS:

- Assorted veggies (bell peppers, zucchini, cherry tomatoes, etc.)
- Olive oil
- Garlic, minced
- Fresh herbs (rosemary, thyme, oregano), chopped
- Salt and pepper

PREPARATION METHOD:

1. Preheat oven to 425°F (220°C).
2. Toss different veggies with olive oil, minced garlic, chopped fresh herbs, salt, and pepper.
3. Spread the veggies on a baking sheet.
4. Roast for 20-25 minutes or until veggies are brown and soft.

10. Cauliflower Rice Stir-Fry with Shrimp

INTRODUCTION:

A low-carb option that doesn't sacrifice on taste. Cauliflower rice, stir-fried with luscious shrimp and an assortment of veggies, offers a heart-healthy and tasty supper.

INGREDIENTS:

- Cauliflower, riced
- Shrimp, peeled and deveined
- Broccoli florets
- Bell peppers, sliced
- Soy sauce, low-sodium
- Sesame oil
- Ginger, grated
- Garlic, minced
- Green onions, chopped

PREPARATION METHOD:

1. In a wok, stir-fry shrimp until pink and cooked through.

2. Add riced cauliflower, broccoli, and chopped bell peppers.
3. Mix low-sodium soy sauce, sesame oil, grated ginger, and chopped garlic in a bowl.
4. Pour the sauce over the stir-fry and mix until fully incorporated.
5. Garnish with chopped green onions.

11. Whole Grain Pasta with Tomato-Basil Sauce

INTRODUCTION:
A heart-healthy take on a classic. Whole grain pasta coupled with a handmade tomato-basil sauce, incorporating antioxidant-rich tomatoes and fragrant basil.

INGREDIENTS:
- Whole grain pasta
- Tomatoes, diced
- Fresh basil, chopped

- Olive oil
- Garlic, minced
- Red pepper flakes (optional)
- Parmesan cheese, grated
- Salt & pepper

PREPARATION METHOD:
1. Cook whole grain pasta according to package directions.
2. In a skillet, sauté minced garlic in olive oil until aromatic.
3. Add chopped tomatoes and simmer until softened.
4. Stir in chopped fresh basil, red pepper flakes (if using), salt, and pepper.
5. Toss the cooked pasta in the tomato-basil sauce.
6. Serve topped with grated Parmesan cheese.

12. Chia Seed Pudding with Berries

INTRODUCTION:

A heart-healthy dessert or breakfast alternative using chia seeds, famed for their omega-3 fatty acids. Topped with fresh berries for additional antioxidants.

INGREDIENTS:

- Chia seeds
- Almond milk, unsweetened
- Vanilla extract
- Maple syrup
- Mixed berries (strawberries, blueberries, raspberries)

PREPARATION METHOD:

1. Mix chia seeds, unsweetened almond milk, vanilla extract, and maple syrup in a bowl.

2. Stir thoroughly and refrigerate for at least 2 hours or overnight until the liquid thickens.

3. Serve the chia seed pudding topped with mixed berries.

13. Turkey and Vegetable Skewers

INTRODUCTION:

Protein-packed turkey skewers with a rainbow of veggies. Grilled to perfection, these skewers provide a heart-healthy alternative to standard meat selections.

INGREDIENTS:

- Ground turkey
- Bell peppers (assorted colors), sliced into bits
- Cherry tomatoes
- Red onion, sliced into wedges
- Olive oil
- Italian seasoning

- Garlic powder
- Salt and pepper

PREPARATION METHOD:
1. Preheat the grill or grill pan.
2. In a bowl, combine ground turkey with olive oil, Italian seasoning, garlic powder, salt, and pepper.
3. Form the seasoned turkey mixture into tiny meatballs.
4. Thread meatballs onto skewers, alternating with bits of bell peppers, cherry tomatoes, and red onion.
5. Grill until turkey is cooked through and veggies are browned.

14. Cabbage and Apple Slaw

INTRODUCTION:
A crisp and refreshing slaw that blends the heart-healthy benefits of cabbage with the natural sweetness of apples. The acidic dressing offers a punch of flavor.

INGREDIENTS:

- Green cabbage, thinly sliced
- Red cabbage, thinly sliced
- Apples, julienned
- Greek yogurt
- Dijon mustard
- Apple cider vinegar
- Honey
- Celery seeds
- Salt and pepper

PREPARATION METHOD:

1. In a large dish, add thinly sliced green cabbage, red cabbage, and julienned apples.

2. In a small bowl, mix together Greek yogurt, Dijon mustard, apple cider vinegar, honey, celery seeds, salt, and pepper.

3. Pour the dressing over the cabbage and apple combination.

4. Toss until nicely coated.

15. Sardine and Avocado Whole Grain Wrap

INTRODUCTION:

A omega-3-rich wrap combining sardines and creamy avocado. Whole grain wrap contains fiber, making it a heart-healthy and fulfilling lunch alternative.

INGREDIENTS:

- Whole grain wraps
- Sardines in olive oil, drained
- Avocado, sliced
- Cherry tomatoes, halved
- Red onion, thinly sliced
- Fresh cilantro, chopped
- Lime juice
- Salt and pepper

PREPARATION METHOD:

1. Lay out whole grain wrappers.

2. Place sardines, avocado slices, cherry tomatoes, and thinly sliced red onion on each roll.

3. Sprinkle chopped fresh cilantro over the ingredients.

4. Drizzle lime juice over the fillings.

5. Season with salt and pepper.

6. Roll the wrappers and fasten with toothpicks if required.

16. Eggplant and Chickpea Curry

INTRODUCTION:
A tasty and heart-healthy curry containing eggplant and protein-packed chickpeas. This plant-based cuisine is rich in antioxidants and spices.

INGREDIENTS:
- Eggplant, cubed
- Chickpeas, canned and washed
- Tomatoes, diced

- Onion, finely chopped
- Garlic, minced
- Ginger, grated
- Curry powder
- Cumin, ground
- Coriander, ground
- Coconut milk, light
- Olive oil
- Fresh cilantro, chopped
- Salt & pepper

PREPARATION METHOD:

1. In a skillet, sauté chopped onion, minced garlic, and grated ginger in olive oil until softened.

2. Add diced eggplant and heat until slightly browned.

3. Stir in diced tomatoes, chickpeas, curry powder, powdered cumin, ground coriander, salt, and pepper.

4. Pour in light coconut milk and let the curry boil until eggplant is soft.

5. Garnish with chopped fresh cilantro before serving.

17. Mango and Avocado Salsa with Grilled Chicken

INTRODUCTION:

A delicious and heart-healthy salsa combining the exotic flavors of mango and creamy avocado. Paired with grilled chicken, it's a lovely and healthful lunch.

INGREDIENTS:

- Grilled chicken breasts
- Mango, diced
- Avocado, diced
- Red onion, finely chopped
- Jalapeño, minced
- Lime juice
- Fresh cilantro, chopped
- Salt & pepper

PREPARATION METHOD:

1. Grill chicken breasts until cooked through.

2. In a bowl, add diced mango, diced avocado, finely sliced red onion, minced jalapeño, lime juice, chopped fresh cilantro, salt, and pepper.

3. Serve grilled chicken topped with mango and avocado salsa.

18. Broiled Cod with Lemon and Garlic

INTRODUCTION:

A light and heart-healthy choice with fish fillets grilled to perfection with tangy lemon and garlic. High in protein and low in saturated fat.

INGREDIENTS:

- Cod fillets
- Fresh lemon juice
- Garlic, minced
- Olive oil
- Paprika
- Fresh parsley, chopped
- Salt & pepper

PREPARATION METHOD:

1. Preheat the broiler.

2. Place fish fillets on a baking sheet.

3. Mix fresh lemon juice, minced garlic, olive oil, paprika, chopped fresh parsley, salt, and pepper in a basin.

4. Brush the lemon-garlic mixture over the fish fillets.

5. Broil for 8-10 minutes or until the salmon flakes easily.

19. Spaghetti Squash with Tomato-Basil Sauce

INTRODUCTION:

A nutritious and low-carb alternative to regular spaghetti. Spaghetti squash strands mixed with a homemade tomato-basil sauce for a heart-healthy and tasty supper.

INGREDIENTS:

- Spaghetti squash, halves and seeds removed
- Tomatoes, diced
- Fresh basil, chopped
- Garlic, minced
- Olive oil
- Balsamic vinegar
- Red pepper flakes (optional)
- Parmesan cheese, grated
- Salt & pepper

PREPARATION METHOD:

1. Preheat the oven to 375°F (190°C).
2. Place spaghetti squash halves on a baking sheet, cut side down.
3. Roast for 40-45 minutes or until the squash is soft.
4. In a skillet, sauté chopped garlic in olive oil until aromatic.
5. Add diced tomatoes, chopped fresh basil, balsamic vinegar, red pepper flakes (if using), salt, and pepper.

6. Scrape the spaghetti squash with a fork to produce strands.

7. Toss the strands in the tomato-basil sauce.

8. Serve topped with grated Parmesan cheese.

20. Berry and Yogurt Parfait

INTRODUCTION:

A delectable and heart-healthy parfait containing layers of Greek yogurt and juicy berries. Packed with antioxidants, it's a guilt-free dessert or brunch alternative.

INGREDIENTS:

- Greek yogurt
- Mixed berries (strawberries, blueberries, raspberries)
- Granola
- Honey

PREPARATION METHOD:

1. In a glass or dish, layer Greek yogurt.
2. Add a layer of mixed berries.
3. Sprinkle granola over the berries.
4. Repeat the layers until the glass or bowl is full.
5. Drizzle honey over the top.
6. Serve this Berry and Yogurt Parfait cold.

Conclusion

In the magnificent symphony of life, the "Heart Disease Diet Cookbook for Seniors" appears as a conductor, orchestrating a crescendo of energy and well-being. As we end this culinary chapter, remember: this cookbook is not only a collection of dishes; it's a lifeline to heart health. With each meticulously created meal, it has become a compass, directing elders toward a symphony of tastes that harmonize with cardiovascular wellbeing.

In the kitchen, this cookbook is more than pages; it's a manifesto, converting meals into rituals of healing and resilience. The quest to manage and win over heart disease is a deep one, and this cookbook is a true companion on that walk. It's about tasting not just the nutrients but reveling in the process of fueling oneself.

So, here's to many years filled with heart-healthy choices, to culinary excursions that embrace well-being, and to seniors who have accepted this cookbook as a protector of their heart's symphony. As the last page flips, may it be a precursor to a life full in flavor, vitality, and the eternal beat of a heart well-cared for. Bon appétit to a heart-healthy future!

Contact Us

Dear valued reader,

First and foremost, I would like to express my sincere gratitude for choosing my book **HEART DISEASE DIET COOKBOOK FOR SENIORS** as your guide. I hope that you found the content helpful, informative, and enjoyable to read.

The Bonus - Special Meal Journal is in the next page.

I also want to remind you that your feedback is important to me. I would love to hear your thoughts, observations, questions and suggestions about the book, so that I can continue to improve and provide you with even more valuable content in the future.

You can contact me through this email: Rebeccahelpdesk@gmail.com

Thank you once again for choosing my book, and I look forward to hearing from you soon!

Best regards,
Rebecca Dorron

BONUS - SPECIAL MEAL TRACKER

SPECIAL MEAL TRACKER

DATE:.................................

MONDAY	BREAKFAST	
	LUNCH	
	DINNER	
TUESDAY	BREAKFAST	
	LUNCH	
	DINNER	
WEDNESDAY	BREAKFAST	
	LUNCH	
	DINNER	
THURSDAY	BREAKFAST	
	LUNCH	
	DINNER	
FRIDAY	BREAKFAST	
	LUNCH	
	DINNER	
SATURDAY	BREAKFAST	
	LUNCH	
	DINNER	
SUNDAY	BREAKFAST	
	LUNCH	
	DINNER	

SNACKS

NOTE

SPECIAL MEAL TRACKER

DATE:................................

MONDAY	BREAKFAST	
	LUNCH	
	DINNER	
TUESDAY	BREAKFAST	
	LUNCH	
	DINNER	
WEDNESDAY	BREAKFAST	
	LUNCH	
	DINNER	
THURSDAY	BREAKFAST	
	LUNCH	
	DINNER	
FRIDAY	BREAKFAST	
	LUNCH	
	DINNER	
SATURDAY	BREAKFAST	
	LUNCH	
	DINNER	
SUNDAY	BREAKFAST	
	LUNCH	
	DINNER	

SNACKS

NOTE

SPECIAL MEAL TRACKER

DATE:..................................

MONDAY	BREAKFAST	
	LUNCH	
	DINNER	
TUESDAY	BREAKFAST	
	LUNCH	
	DINNER	
WEDNESDAY	BREAKFAST	
	LUNCH	
	DINNER	
THURSDAY	BREAKFAST	
	LUNCH	
	DINNER	
FRIDAY	BREAKFAST	
	LUNCH	
	DINNER	
SATURDAY	BREAKFAST	
	LUNCH	
	DINNER	
SUNDAY	BREAKFAST	
	LUNCH	
	DINNER	

SNACKS

NOTE

SPECIAL MEAL TRACKER

DATE:..............................

			SNACKS
MONDAY	BREAKFAST		
	LUNCH		
	DINNER		
TUESDAY	BREAKFAST		
	LUNCH		
	DINNER		
WEDNESDAY	BREAKFAST		
	LUNCH		
	DINNER		
THURSDAY	BREAKFAST		
	LUNCH		
	DINNER		
FRIDAY	BREAKFAST		NOTE
	LUNCH		
	DINNER		
SATURDAY	BREAKFAST		
	LUNCH		
	DINNER		
SUNDAY	BREAKFAST		
	LUNCH		
	DINNER		

SPECIAL MEAL TRACKER

DATE:.................................

MONDAY	BREAKFAST	
	LUNCH	
	DINNER	
TUESDAY	BREAKFAST	
	LUNCH	
	DINNER	
WEDNESDAY	BREAKFAST	
	LUNCH	
	DINNER	
THURSDAY	BREAKFAST	
	LUNCH	
	DINNER	
FRIDAY	BREAKFAST	
	LUNCH	
	DINNER	
SATURDAY	BREAKFAST	
	LUNCH	
	DINNER	
SUNDAY	BREAKFAST	
	LUNCH	
	DINNER	

SNACKS

NOTE

SPECIAL MEAL TRACKER

DATE:....................................

			SNACKS
MONDAY	BREAKFAST		
	LUNCH		
	DINNER		
TUESDAY	BREAKFAST		
	LUNCH		
	DINNER		
WEDNESDAY	BREAKFAST		
	LUNCH		
	DINNER		
THURSDAY	BREAKFAST		
	LUNCH		
	DINNER		
FRIDAY	BREAKFAST		NOTE
	LUNCH		
	DINNER		
SATURDAY	BREAKFAST		
	LUNCH		
	DINNER		
SUNDAY	BREAKFAST		
	LUNCH		
	DINNER		